Life Subject To Change

L. Anne Carrington

Palm Tree Books

Tampa

Dedicated to my readers who took initiatives to improve their respective qualities of life by means of preventive care.

Books by L. Anne Carrington

The Cruiserweight Series:

The Cruiserweight
The Cruiserweight's Daughter
Klass Act
The Marilyn Diaries

Other Fiction:

Fifty

Nonfiction:

Life Subject To Change

Contents

Author's Note

The inspiration behind writing *Life Subject To Change* came after I received what first appeared to be disturbing results of a routine medical test during the late summer of 2013. I was always consistent far as annual routine physicals and gynecological exams went, but often lapsed on other preventive measures until something went wrong or I grew tired of hearing my doctor's office recommend certain tests.

Using my skills as an author and freelance journalist, I made use of available resources - physicians, nurses, personal medical records, death certificates, family history, and information from non-profit health organizations to gather information you'll find in this book.

I neither work in nor have any affiliations with the medical system. I only speak from personal experience with goals to offer readers insights into not taking one's health for granted - no matter how well you feel - and continue seeking answers if an initial diagnosis doesn't seem right.

We only have one chance on this earth and owe it to ourselves to take advantage of opportunities to live full lives as possible. I wish everyone a New Year filled with happiness, success, and robust health.

L. Anne Carrington
January   *2014*

"Is That Really Necessary?"

"An ounce of prevention is worth a pound of cure."
- Benjamin Franklin

More than one million people in the United States are diagnosed with some form of cancer each year. With such numbers, it's astonishing how many options for successful long-term treatment or survival are still diminished because some patients either don't partake in preventive screenings recommended by primary care physicians (PCP's) or seek follow-up care.

I was one of those procrastinators for almost a year. While family history of cancer ran strong, I scoffed at my doctor's advice of having specific screenings done when I reached middle age.

When Dr. Rudolph Antoncic strongly recommended a mammogram during my 2012 annual physical, I wondered if he'd taken leave of his senses.

"Is that really necessary?" I asked. "I've done self-exams every month since I was eighteen."

I was indeed doing the right thing all those years, but soon learned not all abnormalities are detected through breast self-examinations (BSE's) alone.

He stressed the importance of having a mammogram done to catch anything possibly missed during my monthly BSE.

I often heard stories about painful mammograms; some women reported bruising not long after their own procedures. With my general low tolerance of pain and tendency to bruise easily, such horror stories further shut off my ears to Dr. Antoncic's recommendations.

According to the United States Preventive Services Task Force, women between the ages of 50 and 75 are advised to have a mammogram every one to two years, a change from the previous ages of 40 and over. The recommended ages were increased after new evidence revealed screening women between 40 and 50 probably did not save many lives and only exposed women to unneeded radiation from mammograms.

In any case, several physicians suggest their patients be screened at age 40, particularly if there are close family members diagnosed and treated for breast cancer.

Some women young as their thirties have had mammograms; however, they aren't effective screening tools since breasts in women under age 50 are too dense for mammograms to distinguish concerning masses.

Even after learning the aforementioned information, I still refused to have a mammogram. There's no breast cancer history in my family of which I'm aware, and what was the point of wasting time, pain, and money on something that would likely produce a normal result anyway?

Ridiculous...right?

Wrong.

Nevertheless, I kept blowing off mammogram appointments several times for almost a year.

What eventually changed my mind?

I received yet another phone call from his office concerning getting a mammogram. Realizing they weren't going to let the issue go, I caved in and scheduled an appointment; not for health reasons - at least initially - but to shut up everyone for the time being.

I'd like to think continued nagging by Dr. Antoncic and his physician's assistant made me cave, but looking back, the latter were only minor factors in reconsidering my prior resistance to having what I now consider an important test.

Not long after scheduling the appointment, I discovered one of my sisters succumbed to ovarian cancer less than two months shy of her fifty-eighth birthday.

Learning about her death affected me though I hadn't seen her for many years. Past history indicated she likely wasn't diligent in receiving proper medical testing whether or not warranted until it was too late. In our household, going to the doctor and having preventive screenings wasn't done "unless necessary."

Unfortunately for Janice and our parents, such beliefs eventually cost them their lives.

I decided not make the same mistake if I wanted to live to at least age 70 - something neither my sister nor parents had opportunities to do - I needed to take control of my health.

I became determined to not again cancel my mammogram appointment and prepare for whatever results it produced, the fear of pain and bruises be damned!

***

August 6, 2013

This machine was created by a man,
Of this, I have no doubt.
I'd like to stick his balls in there,
And see how THEY come out!
- Excerpt from Julia Napier's poem *The Mammogram*

I arrived at UPMC McKeesport afternoon of August 6 wondering if keeping my appointment was such a good idea. On top of the pain I expected to endure, not wearing antiperspirant as instructed on the notice received a week before my appointment made me self-conscious and I was anxious about getting lost.

However, nothing stopped me. I wasn't getting any younger and had plenty of living left to do.

Once I registered at the front desk and was sent upstairs to where my mammogram took place, my initial fears and concerns dissipated when a mammographer explained the procedure and estimated how long it would take.

The mammographer advised I would receive a phone call and/or written notice if the mammogram results displayed anything of concern. Such practices are common with first-time mammograms since doctors have no previous results in which to compare findings.

Everything got underway after a less than ten-minute wait, the first of a few somewhat pleasant surprises.

The machine appeared less intimidating than imagined. I had to stand for a specific period of time, which posed another concern - least at first - since I have severe osteoarthritis in both knees, but ended up having no problems in that respect.

Sensations felt during the actual mammogram were more mild pressure/tugging than pain and I never noticed any bruising either following the test or days afterward.

Six images of each breast were completed in little over fifteen minutes. I felt like a fool for putting off past appointments and wasting valuable time with worries over minor things for almost a year.

While having a mammogram isn't something I'd put at the top of a list of favorite things to do, it wasn't terrifying as I originally thought.

8

For anyone who hesitated having one done as I initially had, I can't stress enough that catching any abnormalities in its early stages is worth going through some discomfort.

I walked out of the hospital confident everything would be all right and wouldn't need to schedule another mammogram for another two years.

You know what they say about the word 'assume'...

***

(Un)expected Results

"But life inevitably throws us curve balls, unexpected circumstances that remind us to expect the unexpected. I've come to understand these curve balls are the beautiful unfolding of both karma and current." - Carre Otis

My entire day was planned when I woke up the morning of August 9; a deadline for my latest novel was drawing near and the manuscript needed additional work.

I considered shutting off both my land line and cell phones to avoid interruptions while I worked, but my partner was due to return that afternoon from Tampa. He always liked to check in with me after arriving so I knew he safely arrived home.

Most of the morning was spent engrossed in Herculean tasks of writing, rewriting, and editing before I took a one o'clock lunch break.

I assumed Don's plane was en route to Pittsburgh since I still hadn't heard from him, so I didn't bother glimpsing at the Caller ID when the phone on my desk rang.

It wasn't the call I'd been expecting.

A woman identified herself as a UPMC McKeesport Nurse Navigator and informed me that my mammogram had shown some abnormalities. I needed to schedule follow-up tests soon as possible.

I had no initial concerns, I only thought the doctor found something along the lines of shadows and wanted to rule out something more serious.

Despite being warned by the radiologist about a possible telephone call and/or letter before my initial mammogram, she never mentioned anything about an ultrasound.

I drew in a deep, shuddering breath. *Oh, God; this can't be good.*

My follow-up test was set for September 4. The nurse navigator then informed me more detailed results of the first mammogram would be sent to my HealthTrak account.

Don called minutes after I finished my conversation with the nurse navigator.

"Your timing couldn't be any better," I said.

"What's the matter? You sound stressed."

I told him about the abnormal results, adding I had an appointment in early September for additional testing.

"Yeah, they warned you during your first appointment something like this might happen."

"Nobody informed me I'd also need an ultrasound!"

"You shouldn't worry until you know exactly what's happening, Lori. The doctor probably wants further studies on something unusual he'd seen. Don't shrug off this appointment. You should follow through on the September appointment."

"Easy for you to say; you're not having a second round of boobie squashing."

"You have little reason to freak out. Get more information; Google's your friend. If a serious problem does show up on the new test, it's likely to be caught early and you'll be okay."

"I suppose there's no better time to start than check out the first report once they email it."

"Let me know if you find anything interesting. I'll be home in about an hour."

***

I sifted through the day's mail after talking with Don and spotted a letter from UPMC McKeesport's radiology department among the ubiquitous amount of junk mail and household bills.

The letter stated nothing different from what the nurse navigator relayed during our phone conversation.

Disgusted, I checked the HealthTrak account. One unread message waited:

You have new information.

I held my breath and clicked on the link that led to a site displaying the August 6 mammogram results.

When I opened the page, it didn't take long for me to discover a reason behind the urgency to return for an ultrasound and second mammogram.

MAMMOGRAM DIGITAL SCREENING BILATERAL W/ CAD

CLINICAL HISTORY:
Screening.

COMPARISON:
Today's Study is the patient's baseline.

TECHNIQUE:
Full-field digital mammography of the right and left breasts was performed in the CC and MLO projections with CAD. In addition, a lateral exaggerated CC projection of the left breast was obtained.

FINDINGS:
There are scattered fibroglandular densities (approximately 25-50% glandular). Along the left breast upper-outer quadrant, there is an isodense nodule. Along the right breast upper and outer quadrant, there are is a small cluster of indeterminate microcalcifications. There are multiple other benign appearing calcifications throughout both breasts. There are no other significant abnormalities.

IMPRESSION:
. Indeterminate left breast upper and outer quadrant nodule.

. Indeterminate right breast upper-outer quadrant clustered microcalcifications.

OVERALL ASSESSMENT:
BI-RADS CATEGORY 0- Needs Further Imaging Evaluation.

RECOMMENDATIONS:
Additional mammographic views and/or sonography are recommended within 1 month.The UPMC McKeesport Nurse Navigator will coordinate follow up care.

I researched terminologies outlined above in order to explain them in much layman's language as possible.

Most computer-aided detection (CAD) mammographies are limited to single views; however, radiologists are now trained to judge and combine different views, which may explain why so many "pictures" are taken when we have mammograms done. The average number of films taken during mammograms is four, but can vary from patient to patient.

Radiologists can make comparisons between patterns in left and right breasts. In mammography, it's common to make a medio lateral oblique (MLO, the most important projection as it allows depicting most breast tissue) and craniocaudal (CC, showing medial and external lateral portions of the breast).

When the former and latter are independently viewed, abnormalities are often marked in one view despite appearing visually similar since differences in features computed in the two views may cause considerable differences in lesions assigned by the CAD procedure.

Scattered fibroglandular densities can sound confusing and nerve-racking to the average person, but this is basically a form of breast tissue density identification. A woman's breasts are composed of glandular tissue, fibrous connective tissue and fat.

Fibroglandular breast tissue includes the milk ducts in the breast and the fibers that support the breast.

The Breast Imaging Reporting and Data System (BI-RADS) classifications identify four levels of breast density, keeping with relative increases in the amount of levels of fibro-glandular tissue:

Type 1: Breast density is almost entirely fat; glandular tissue is less than 25 percent.

Type 2 (this type was outlined in my report): Scattered fibroglandular tissues are present, which range from 25 to 50 percent of the breast.

Type 3: This classification is 'heterogeneously dense', ranging 51 to 75 percent of breast tissue.

'Heterogeneous' means something contains many different items and variations. With respect to breast density, it implies fibrous tissue is prevalent throughout the breast yet not clustered together.

Type 4: The highest BI-RAD category of breast density, containing greater than 75 percent glandular and fibrous tissue. The sensitivity of mammograms may be reduced in Level 4 breast density.

'Indeterminate microcalcifications' is another term that can first appear unsettling to patients - including me - until we learn its meaning.

Basically speaking, indeterminate microcalcifications difficult to classify are often labeled indeterminate. They are specks of calcium found in areas of rapidly dividing cells and appear as microcalcifications from residue left by rapidly dividing cells. When microcalcifications are seen in a cluster, they may indicate small cancers. Approximately half these cancers appear in clusters.

The term 'microcalcification' is often used for calcifications found with malignancy, usually smaller, more numerous, clustered, and variously shaped (rods, branches, teardrops). Calcifications associated with benign conditions are usually larger, fewer in number, widely dispersed, and round.

There is good news amidst all this information: the majority of breast calcifications are non-cancerous. What those calcifications actually are remain a mystery and vary from woman to woman, but it never hurts to take precautions in case something is amiss.

On a side note, these calcifications should not be confused with calcium found in dairy products. All the milk we drink has nothing to do with those little deposits turning up in a mammogram.

The isodense nodule noted in my results is sometimes moderately suspicious of malignancy, another factor which could've weighed in me having a second study done.

In conclusion, it appeared the doctor was most concerned about the nodule and the microcalfication clusters, since tight clusters of tiny calcifications can indicate breast cancer.

Don was right about one thing; gleaning more information about the current test results did bring some peace of mind. I still had some anxiety about my upcoming appointment but no intentions of skipping it.

Better safe than sorry.

***

September 4, 2013

"Mammograms are really sort of a gift. You can either catch something early or count your lucky stars because nothing was discovered. Either way, you're ahead of the game."
- Charlotte Ross

"Want me to come along and hold your hand?" Don asked during breakfast.

"If you're trying to be funny, it isn't working," I replied. "They probably won't let you back in the test area anyway."

"I'm serious; even reassured by all the online reading you've done, I can tell you're still nervous. That's why I took a day off from work. I have plenty of people to keep an eye on my businesses."

I couldn't help but smile at his kind gesture. "Thanks, it'll be great to have someone with me this time."

"What time is your appointment?"

"One o'clock, but I have to be registered at least fifteen minutes prior to it."

"We'll leave between quarter after twelve and twelve-thirty. Do you know anything about hospital parking?"

"There's a lot by the emergency room and a visitor garage, but I have no idea what they cost."

"I'll figure out something. Don't forget to pack deodorant in your purse to put on afterward. Much as I love you, armpit odor lingering in my car hardly sounds delectable."

"Very funny, Don. I'm way ahead of you."

"Why *can't* you use any?"

"Most deodorants and body powders contain aluminum."

"So?"

"From what the scheduling nurse told me before I had the first mammogram, aluminum in deodorant and powder looks similar to breast calcifications and can hamper seeing authentic ones while reading mammograms. God knows I already have enough calcifications without doing something to make the new tests look worse than they actually are."

"Nothing's getting worse. I have a feeling the outcome will be great."

"Would you think the same if your 'boys' were the ones being twisted in several directions and flattened a second time?"

"Probably not, but I thought you said the first test wasn't painful."

"No, but there's little guarantee I'll have the same mammographer. She really knew her stuff."

"I'm sure you'll get someone else who also knows what they're doing. At least we know the ultrasound will be painless."

"Yeah, but we aren't getting anything accomplished sitting and talking. It's already after eleven and I need to shower before we leave."

***

I wasn't nervous about the second mammogram since I now knew what to expect.

The waiting room was busier than my last visit; four women were scheduled ahead of me. I didn't mind since Don and I arrived earlier than expected, cutting out need to rush in the dressing area before my mammogram.

Having Don along helped a great deal. I not only had someone to distract my mind from what lay ahead, but also didn't need to worry how long I'd have to wait for a bus home.

A different person performed my mammogram as expected. She was also knowledgeable about the procedure and I again felt more pressure than pain.

Once the mammogram was completed, my next step was having an ultrasound.

A doctor worked with the radiologist concentrating on further studies of my microcalcifications and isodense nodule. Since the majority of abnormalities appeared in my left breast, I was instructed to lie on my right side with a foam rubber block placed behind me.

Unlike mammograms, breast (and other) ultrasound procedures don't use radiation, therefore posing no risk to patients.

These types of ultrasounds determine whether abnormalities detected in a mammography or palpable lumps are fluid-filled cysts or solid tumors, and if they're malignant or benign.

Breast ultrasounds are generally not used as screening tools for cancer detection because they do not always detect early signs such as microcalcifications. While a further study on clustered microcalcifications was warranted in my case, my guess turned out correct that greater concerns concentrated on the nodule.

The entire ultrasound took less than twenty minutes. I dressed while the doctor was out of the room to read my test results. I didn't wait long before he and the radiologist returned with a good report.

All findings turned up *benign* results!

Copies of both the ultrasound and second mammogram would be sent to my HealthTrak account, but the radiologist handed me a sheet briefly outlining their findings.

To say I was relieved to hear such news was an understatement; I all but floated out of the ultrasound lab.

"Don't tell me," Don said when I returned to the waiting room. "Everything went well."

"How did you guess?" I asked with a broad smile on my face.

"See? You did all that worrying about nothing."

"Don't get carried away with gloating, mister. I have to return for another mammogram next September."

"I thought you only needed one every two years."

"Wow, someone's been catching up on his reading. Two years is an estimate, but once a year is recommended for anyone with a prior abnormal mammogram."

I waved the sheet in my hand. "If I keep getting results like these, I won't mind having my girls flattened and twisted once a year. Believe me; something far worse may have been avoided these past several weeks."

***

A longer outline of my results arrived two days later. I had a general idea what they meant without looking up most definitions appearing in my copy of the report.

Throughout my mammogram experience, I'd become familiar with terms such as BI-RAD, microcalcifications, isodense nodules, various types of breast densities, milk of calcium, and benign etiology among others.

The second results' page gave me little different information in contrast to what I was told at the hospital; only difference was the following results are more detailed.

US BREAST BILATERAL - Details

CLINICAL HISTORY:
Asymptomatic 51-year-old female recalled from her recent baseline mammogram for a left breast nodule and right breast microcalcifications.

DIAGNOSTIC BILATERAL BREAST MAMMOGRAM:
Digital magnification mammography of the right breast was performed in the CC and ML projections. Spot compression views of the left breast were obtained in the CC and MLO projection. Comparison is made to the patient's baseline mammogram dated August 6, 2013.

The previously noted right breast upper and outer quadrant clustered microcalcifications are noted to be associated with milk of calcium consistent with a benign etiology. The left breast upper and outer quadrant nodule is ovoid, fat containing, dense, and has partially obscured margins. It will be further evaluated sonographically.

LEFT BREAST SONOGRAM:
Multiple transverse and longitudinal targeted sonographic images of the upper and outer quadrant of the left breast were obtained. Between the 1 and 2 o'clock positions, there is a ovoid mixed echo nodule with cystic and fatty changes corresponding to the mammographic nodule in question. This is most consistent with an incidental hamartoma. Between the 12 and 1 o'clock positions, a subcentimeter thinly septated cyst was incidentally noted. No other abnormalities were appreciated.

IMPRESSION:
. No mammographic evidence of malignancy in the right breast.

. No mammographic or sonographic evidence of malignancy in the left breast.

OVERALL ASSESSMENT:
BI-RADS Category 2- Benign findings

RECOMMENDATIONS:
The patient may now return to her annual screening mammography schedule.

The patient was given a written and verbal summary of the above findings and recommendations.

Not intimidating as the first set of results, though a few new terms appeared on the new reading.

Ovoid mixed echo nodule is basically nothing more than another name for a benign nodule, and cysts are the most common types of masses.

"Milk of calcium" can sound a bit confusing, but not the same as a jug of white fluid sitting in our refrigerators. Milk of calcium in reference to breast imaging studies is a reassuring term for the vast majority of benign results.

Incidental hamartoma is one of few breast abnormalities with characteristic features that allow confident diagnosis without resort to needle biopsy or surgical excision. If this description turns up in any test results, one can feel somewhat assured a needle biopsy or worse is unlikely to follow.

I'll sum up in layman's terms and say with confidence that I not only dodged one bullet, but *two*...at least for now. My next mammogram is due September 2014, and I have zero intentions of missing that appointment. One scare was more than enough for me.

***

Why Continuing Family Tradition Isn't Always Wise

"If we can make the correct diagnosis, the healing can begin. If we can't, both our personal health and our economy are doomed."
- Andrew Weil

I often joked that I was healthy before everything began going to hell after age thirty. In truth, everything unraveled during my late twenties with gradually diminished hearing and mysterious fainting spells.

It didn't matter if I sat, stood, took a casual stroll around the neighborhood, or just went through my workday; there were no indications as to when or why I'd lose consciousness.

Countless visits to medical professionals provided virtually nil results. I received diagnoses from orthostatic hypotension, vasovagal syncope, stress, and my favorite - coming from a person who was my therapist at the time - "psychosomatic reactions to unresolved issues."

I'd spend years seeking every feasible treatment for a condition that left medical professionals scratching their heads in bemusement to the point of grudgingly accepting fainting without prior warning as part of my existence.

Now I knew why my parents didn't visit doctors often and rarely took us kids unless they deemed it necessary despite my father having excellent insurance coverage through his job. Unfortunately for all involved, their decisions far as health care was concerned weren't always the right ones.

***

My siblings and I had healthy childhoods, but at least one consequence of my parents' views of regular medical care remains with me to the present day.

I developed ear infections in my early teens treated at home with drops of sweet oil (also known as olive oil in some cases) placed in my ears and stuffed with cotton. The ear infections eventually cleared up, but the extent of damage to my hearing wasn't uncovered for another two decades.

The infections' exact causes were never determined since I never saw a doctor. I started noticing changes in my ears and hearing - albeit minor at first - during my twenties. Certain word sounds became more difficult to distinguish; I could barely hear medium-frequency noises and no low-frequency ones in my right ear, though high-frequency sounds   remained   clear.

I kept my hearing limitations hidden by becoming proficient in lip reading and positioned myself so others could speak into my left ear when unable to altogether avoid conversations.

I attended a health fair where free hearing tests were offered among other health screenings. I took advantage on a whim, not expecting less than normal results for someone my age. The volunteer audiologist stated I not only had 40 percent loss of hearing in my right ear, but also 10 percent loss in the left. She then referred me to another audiology practice for additional tests, all covered by insurance.

The health fair booth findings were confirmed during my first appointment with Mark Gustina at Cranberry Hearing and Balance. I was in no danger of going completely deaf, but had enough substantial loss to warrant being fitted for an aid. Improperly treated ear infections indeed played a role in my hearing issues.

I now wear a hearing device in my right ear which considerably improved my quality of life. I still read lips on occasion, but it's a blessing to no longer yell at people for "mumbling," stand or sit so people are forced to speak into my left ear, and turn up the TV to scream level.

***

When my constant fainting began a few years after I initially noticed ear changes, I wondered if someone missed some inner-ear imbalance problem. My theories were once again dismissed.

The mysteries behind my syncope episodes were unveiled during the summer of 1997 after I passed out twice in a twenty-four hour period.

I was fortunate to have an attending ER physician who cared enough to examine me beyond blood tests, taking blood pressure, tapping joints with a little mallet, squeezing hands, and a "follow my finger with your eyes" routine. He found my complex fainting history unsettling and wouldn't discharge me until he reached a solid diagnosis.

My blood work and actual exam showed normal findings, but the ER doctor wasn't satisfied. He recommended I be admitted to the hospital for further observation and complete workup.

I underwent head MRI's, an EEG, and more blood work the following morning. All tests came back normal with a preliminary diagnosis of idiopathic seizure disorder noted in my records.

Nevertheless, a cardiology consult was ordered.

I met Dr. John Paulowski on my second full day of hospitalization, a physician board certified in cardiology and cardiovascular disease who'd oversee the day's scheduled tests: a stress test with adenosine injection, thallium heart scan, an echocardiogram, and cardiac catheterization.

I was grateful for a medical team dedicated to discovering exact origins to my losses of consciousness, yet I couldn't understand why cardiac tests were needed. Nothing unusual stood out on the emergency room EKG nor was I aware of any prior heart problems.

Dr. Paulowski and his associates finally found answers that eluded me for almost a decade.

No artery blockages turned up during the echocardiogram or catheterization, but signs of cardiomyopathy appeared in the results of my catheterization.

Dr. Paulowski couldn't explain which type I had, so my cardiomyopathy was classified as idiopathic. He reassured me my condition wasn't life-threatening and may be reversible with my continued clean living.

Since I wasn't a smoker, never used street drugs and rarely drank, anything from genetics, viruses, medication side effects and years of yo-yo dieting could've played roles in my condition.

Prinzmetal's angina was discovered in addition to cardiomyopathy. Prinzmetal's is a type of angina caused when coronary arteries narrow by contraction (arterial spasms in layman's terms) rather than atherosclerosis often found in "traditional" angina. The Prinzmetal's diagnosis explained occasional bouts of pain and mild squeezing sensations in my chest I'd often dismissed as indigestion.

After a three-day hospital stay, I was discharged with recommendations to take 325 milligrams of aspirin daily (eventually reduced to 81 milligrams), follow up with the PCP I saw at the time, make a cardiology appointment, and given prescriptions for 300 milligrams of Neurontin and five milligrams of Norvasc.

Neurontin's primary use is treating focal, partial, and mixed seizure disorders, but has been prescribed off label for numbers of conditions including fibromyalgia, chronic neuropathic pain, menopausal symptoms, and itching due to renal failure, to name a few.

Norvasc is a calcium channel blocker prescribed for hypertension (high blood pressure) and effective in treating angina by relaxing the smooth muscle in the arterial wall and increasing blood flow to the heart muscle.

Within weeks of beginning my new regimen, times between fainting became less frequent and altogether ceased the following year.

***

I continued brushing off preventive health care long after treatments for syncope, hearing loss and other issues. Medical procedures and doctors cost money, some not covered by insurance back then.

We all hear stories about seniors and families who make tough decisions between paying bills and for food and receiving proper medical care. There were few occasions where I'd faced similar dilemmas and often cast preventive medicine by the wayside.

I continued to have annual physicals, regular vision and dental exams and took medication but deemed most other preventive measures unnecessary.

I often wonder if my parents and sister would be alive today had they kept closer guard on their health. Some family traditions are fine to continue through generations, but handing down habits shouldn't include neglecting our own well-being.

No amount of money will compensate permanent damage incurred or lives lost as result of not seeking medical attention the moment abnormalities are noticed or even taking opportunities to have something simple as a physical exam.

***

"God Should Issue a Recall On Me!"

*"Can someone find one thing **not** wrong for a change?"*
- Me, September 2005

Those familiar with my extensive medical history probably wonder how I managed to cope with multiple health issues well as I have.

Aside from routine physical and gynecological appointments, I had no contact with the medical community during my younger years until age twenty-one when I was diagnosed with major depressive disorder (MDD) and dysthymia following a suicide attempt.

Overdosing on pills I spotted wasn't the first time I tried to harm myself. The medication ingested wasn't any more fatal than my parents' other prescriptions to which I helped myself during previous attempts; I ended up nauseated and vomiting most of the time.

I was a regular visitor to psychologists' offices during high school - after the guidance counselor's office sent a referral to my parents following what I've since realized was another depressive episode - but none managed to pinpoint origins of my solemn demeanor.

I'm sure they had more than plenty of experience counseling "moody" adolescents and likely disregarded my often-dark state of mind as teen angst; therefore, existing records lacked concrete answers to my condition prior to October 1983.

I had daily consultations with a psychiatrist overseeing my case, but not prescribed medication. She referred me for individual therapy at the city mental health clinic and to a six-month partial hospitalization program.

Both were effective for only a short time.

The next two decades saw me in and out of public and private hospitals, outpatient clinics, temporary residential programs, seeing various psychiatrists and psychologists, being arrested a few times due to many self-destructive behaviors, involved in relationships best described as turbulent, having acupuncture, and taking several types of antidepressants that did little more than cause heartburn, irritability, and drowsiness.

Most pharmacological and talk therapies had scant effect in undermining my symptoms. I'm not against either method; I actually applaud progress made in discovering effective yet less harmful options in treating mental health disorders.

Despite my increased disillusionment with the psychiatric profession, something told me not to give up.

My once-futile efforts started paying off with another round of psychiatric treatment at a prestigious, out of state inpatient center in February 1999.

The supervising psychiatrist speculated that my MDD symptoms could've been resistant to tricyclic antidpressants since Pamelor, Tofranil and Norpramin had failed to provide long term effects.

His initial assessment was confirmed when blood tests revealed below-normal serotonin levels. He prescribed fluoxetine, a selective serotonin reuptake inhibitor (SSRI) known as Prozac among other trade names.

He also replaced my Neurontin with topiramate (brand name Topamax), a drug first approved in the United States in 1996 for treating seizure disorders.

Prozac became my Utopia of sorts; I noticed a considerable improvement within two weeks of starting the SSRI regimen.

While lessening other MDD symptoms, Prozac not only made me feel more energetic and focused, but also brought my then-premenstrual syndrome under control. Topamax decreased my appetite, diminished occasional headaches, and - as I later discovered while researching the medication - could've helped Prozac boost my overall mood.

The psychiatrist also replaced my Neurontin with topriamate, an anticonvulsant to treat certain types of seizures known as Topamax among other brand names.

In addition to its primary use, topiramate is sometimes prescribed "off label" for migraine and cluster headaches, Lennox-Gastaut syndrome (a disorder that causes seizures and developmental delays), alcoholism, essential tremors, obsessive-compulsive disorder, smoking cessation, idiopathic intracranial hypertension, treatment-resistant depression, cocaine and methamphetamine addictions, borderline personality disorder, obesity, binge eating disorder, and bulimia.

When I returned home from what was the last inpatient psychiatric treatment to date, I visited my primary care doctor. He ordered more in-depth blood work and a sleep study in addition to my regular exam.

I returned a week later to discuss test results that had caught his attention.

"Are there any thyroid or respiratory problems in your family?" the doctor asked.

His question baffled me. "One of my sisters had thyroid surgery in the 1970's, I have a niece who had asthma as a child but grew out of it, and my father had emphysema for long as I could remember before he died from lung cancer in 1992. Why?"

"All of other blood work appears fine, but your thyroid level readings were below normal. Your sleep study also turned up patterns related to a milder form of obstructive sleep apnea."

He stressed that in addition to psychological, psychosocial, genetics, and evolutionary factors play roles, often-overlooked physical ailments such as respiratory diseases, sleep disorders, cancer, certain types of heart disease, metabolic imbalances (e.g. diabetes) and long-term substance abuse can also contribute to MDD and dysthymia.

"So you're saying my depression could've been caused by sleep apnea and a sluggish thyroid?" I asked.

"Along with your low serotonin levels and history of cardiomyopathy, but I wouldn't rule out any psychological factors. How long have you been treated for depression?"

"Actively since age twenty-one, but nothing really worked until my last inpatient treatment."

"Sounds like you received effective treatment. The low thyroid function may also contribute to your weight problems. I'll prescribe Synthroid and a 1500-calorie diet. I'll also refer you to a pulmonologist who will further evaluate your sleep apnea and order CPAP therapy."

Positive outcomes emerged from my latest diagnoses: the thyroid and sleep apnea offered reasons behind snoring I was often teased about by well-meaning friends and old roommates, occasional dry skin and swollen ankles and periods of daytime tiredness despite sleeping well (at least I thought).

The CPAP machine and Synthroid eventually balanced out everything in spite of me adjusting to sleeping with a nasal mask clamped to my face every night.

Wearing the mask to bed eventually became second nature; while Don doesn't find it visually appealing on occasions he stays overnight, he understands there are other potential consequences besides his being jarred awake by the sounds of snoring several times a night if I *don't* utilize my CPAP.

Far as my weight is concerned, tendencies to be overweight or obese run rampant among women in my family tree. My maternal great-grandmother allegedly weighed 400 pounds. My maternal grandmother, mother, sisters, and a few nieces struggled with weight troubles.

Genetics and misfiring thyroid aside, I'd dealt with what I eventually viewed as dysfunctional relationships with food from my earliest childhood, but never realized such dysfunction had a name until my last inpatient treatment for depression.

I always loved eating long as I can remember and came from a meat-and-potatoes home where not cleaning one's plate was considered rude. Wasting food was a sin. If a small piece of meat or spoonful of vegetables were left after dinner, they ended up on someone's plate before we left the table. Fast food expeditions were almost unheard of and we rarely ventured to traditional restaurants except for special occasions.

My mother cooked from scratch and I can't recall one time she prepared meals using pre-made ingredients from boxes or cans before the early 1980's when most of us kids already left home.

When I began examining my past relationships with food, I discovered large age gaps between me and most of my siblings (my oldest brother already a teenager when I was born) and what I now realize were emotionally unavailable parents made me feel lonely and contributed to my shyness as a child and adolescent. Beliefs that "proper ladies" didn't publicly express their emotions and psychological disorders being sources of shame didn't help much either.

With all the aforementioned environmental factors, I gained perception that I'd used food as an antidepressant substitute, to avoid dealing with feelings, or dull memories of unpleasant childhood events until they were erased from my mind.

Food was cheaper and more accessible than drugs or alcohol, and stuffing myself to the point of physical discomfort was an easier option than verbally communicating my feelings.

I learned new - and less destructive - coping tools during my last inpatient treatment once I'd begun feeling comfortable enough to openly air my problem with eating.

Something urged me to discuss my eating habits in detail with my designated therapist during one of our individual sessions, a topic I never shared with anyone else.

"What made you bring it up today?" she asked.

"I don't know; maybe because you don't know my family, friends, and co-workers."

"You feel safe."

I nodded. "If other people knew, they'd think I was definitely a head case."

"There's part of your problem," my therapist replied. "You've been conditioned to do for others, value only *their* opinions and base your life on what's socially acceptable. Have you ever asked yourself once what *you* wanted?"

"To be honest, I was rarely encouraged to think for myself because I might have embarrassed my parents or whomever by doing or saying the 'wrong' things."

"What about all emergency room visits because you were suicidal? Didn't you make *those* decisions?"

"Well, yeah; I was still at home my first two admissions to the city hospital's psych ward but living alone or with roommates during following hospitalizations. I received zero support from relatives; one sister actually said I should've gotten the shit beaten out of me 'for the constant pain I caused our parents'."

"I've had patients with family members from different generations who had difficulty grasping their loved ones' major depression diagnosis. They blamed everyone from themselves to the patient's spouse, friends, and the patient. I explained that the patient can live a normal life with proper treatment and no one should be held accountable for their condition."

"I tried that route only to be further mocked," I said. "So I decided it was better to just shut up, avoid everyone, and find other ways to deal with my problems."

"Is overeating one way of coping with unexpressed feelings?"

I nodded. "Too bad my favorite 'coping skill' caused me to gain so much weight."

"Let me ask you a few things. Are you alone during times you eat large quantities, keep eating even after you're full, constantly diet, and often feel guilty after a binge but never purged what you'd eaten?"

Her last questions prompted a light bulb to switch on in my mind. "Yeah, everything you described! How did you know?"

"Are you familiar with something called Binge Eating Disorder?"

"Come on, surely there's no such thing. I came from a family of big eaters; only problem I have is stopping after I'm full."

"Most assume Binge Eating Disorder is only used as an excuse to keep eating when in fact it exists much as anorexia and bulimia. Not all people with BED are overweight or obese. Some patients within normal weight limits have been treated for the disorder."

"I had no idea."

"From what you described and your history of major depression and dysthymic disorders, you have key features of Binge Eating Disorder. You're off to a good start by owning the problem and taking Prozac and Topamax, but I'll talk to the doctor about an outpatient center referral in your area. You should also consider attending Overeaters Anonymous meetings."

I began further reading about Binge Eating Disorder (BED) after returning home and found familiar behaviors listed as symptoms of BED I'd once dismissed as lack of self-control.

The Diagnostic and Statistical Manual of Mental Disorders-IV (DSM-IV) released in 1994 only listed BED in its Appendix B and previously diagnosed patients with BED as EDNOS (Eating Disorder Not Otherwise Specified).

Over one thousand research papers supporting Binge Eating Disorder were published as a specific diagnosis with validity and consistency in the interim, and the release of *DSM-V* by the American Psychiatric Association in May 2013 individually listed Binge Eating Disorder as an actual eating disorder among several additions and modifications made in the *DSM's* current edition.

The outpatient group and Overeater's Anonymous were godsends.

I learned even more about BED, how to pinpoint my "trigger foods," constructive ways to deal with problems other than eating, avoiding toxic people and situations, and most important, letting go of my "stinking thinking."

I took further initiative to enrich my life by participating in local women's empowerment workshops while continuing group therapy and OA meetings.

I no longer felt alone in struggling with a myriad of medical and psychological afflictions; moreover, I received validation of deserving better than what I'd endured for several decades.

***

Despite counseling, OA meetings, empowerment group sessions, extensive reading, and medications playing respective roles in lessening my BED and depressive symptoms, I faced the difficult task of bringing my weight - which teetered near 400 pounds - under control.

I'd lost some weight through working the OA program but considerable amounts of poundage still remained.

My main focus was not looking like a fashion model but avoid additional physical and psychological risks that often accompanied obesity. I was diagnosed with severe knee osteoarthritis in my mid-thirties and didn't want to end up in a wheelchair like my mother did by her fifties.

The thought of losing the smallest iota of hard-won independence unsettled me; I had to take some type of action before arthritis and other health issues were worsened by excess weight I carried.

I considered seeking some type of medical intervention but wasn't sure about available options until reading a newspaper article on weight loss surgery (WLS) in 2004.

Delving further into the article, I found risks of most weight loss surgeries were now much lower than past decades due to less invasive measures like laparoscopic procedures. WLS late as the 1970's required at least a week-long hospital stay whereas WLS is performed today in either same-day surgery centers or an inpatient setting with patients leaving the hospital in little as twenty-four hours.

Let me stress that weight loss surgery is not a cure for obesity nor does all excess weight disappear overnight. This procedure is only a tool; the remaining work depends on us.

I spent many days after reading the newspaper feature searching Pittsburgh area doctors who performed weight loss surgery and noted educational backgrounds, credentials, patient reviews, and hospitals where each performed surgery.

I soon discovered Anita Courcoulas, M.D., M.P.H., F.A.C.S, a board-certified surgeon specializing in bariatric and general surgery with impressive credentials, extensive experience in her specialties, and several pages of positive patient reviews.In addition, she's the University Of Pittsburgh School Of Medicine's Chief of Minimally Invasive Bariatric and General Surgery and a Professor of Surgery.

I spent most of my first appointment's four-hour wait reading additional materials on bariatric surgery, filling out ubiquitous forms, signing releases, and having vital statistics taken.

I knew Dr. Courcoulas was the right doctor for my needs when she came into the exam room and reviewed my medical history in depth. She found me to be an excellent candidate for Roux-en-Y gastric bypass, a procedure which makes the stomach smaller and causes food to bypass part of the small intestine.

For a recovering binger in dire need to lose copious amounts of weight, gastric bypass sounded like an ideal solution.

Pre-surgical preparation took almost a year. Additional medical tests, consultations with a nutritionist, submitting detailed diet and medical histories to my insurance carrier, and undergoing a psychiatric evaluation were ordered between visits to Dr. Courcoulas' office.

I experienced no problems with the medical tests and gathering additional requested information. Dr. Antoncic had become gravely concerned about my skyrocketing weight and supported my decision to have WLS. He forwarded a letter of recommendation to Dr. Courcoulas and the insurance carrier with alacrity.

I didn't look forward to the psych evaluation. I was convinced the examiner would issue a negative report once my history of MDD, dysthymia and binge eating disorder surfaced.

I considered not mentioning anything at all during my evaluation, but not only was I unsure how much the examiner already knew about me, but also coming clean and owning our behaviors often stressed at therapy and Overeaters Anonymous echoed in my brain.

I chose to lay everything in the open, no matter the consequences.

Nothing stood out during my psych evaluation; I was issued the Wechsler Adult Intelligence Scale (WAIS) and Minnesota Multiphasic Personality Inventory (MMPI) tests in addition to discussions on what I expected from gastric bypass surgery and a goal weight. I stressed that I had not binged in almost five years and a solid plan was in place should I have the urges to do so.

I talked about attending OA, my desired goal weight of 150 pounds, and I was aware that weight loss resulting from bariatric surgery would be a gradual process.

A copy of the psych report's contents astonished me. A brief overview of WAIS results showed "a 42-year-old Caucasian female with a Full Scale Score of 122, falling within range of high average to superior range of 116-124."

Further evaluation found I was "aware of potential complication risks during and following elective surgery, well-informed on Roux-en-Y gastric bypass with realistic weight loss goals and strong understanding that WLS is not a permanent cure for morbid obesity."

While the MMPI revealed "marked levels of trust, suspiciousness, sensitivity, and depressive features," apparently the examiner didn't find anything unsettling enough to interfere with her final decision.

I passed the psychiatric evaluation, clearing one more hurdle before surgery would be scheduled. All that remained was my insurance carrier's coverage decision.

***

The first letter I received from my insurance carrier denied coverage for Roux-en-Y gastric bypass due to "insufficient amount of information received" and the surgery being classified as "a cosmetic procedure."

Almost a year's worth of time invested in pre-op preparations down the drain. I was desolate.

I had sixty days to appeal and wasted little time firing off a six-page response as to why the intended surgery was for medical reasons; how the excess weight I carried aggravated the arthritis in my knees, making it difficult to walk more than a block, having constant pain, and how I was considered disabled under specific guidelines due to several medical conditions, deeming me unfit for employment.

I added several promising outcomes of substantial weight loss through bariatric surgery, including increased chances of being medically cleared to seek part-time employment, improvement of mobility and other areas of current health issues, and maintain my independence.

Two more months went by before I received a second letter from my insurance carrier. I was nervous about the envelope's contents as they were far thinner than prior correspondence.

I'm not sure on which desk my appeal landed or what part of its contents inspired someone to overturn the previous decision and approve coverage, but the emotions I felt after reading that letter could only be explained with one word: euphoria.

Surgery took place on September 28, 2005 at UPMC Shadyside. I went into the hospital both nervous and eager to begin a new chapter of my life, optimistic I'd nip my weight difficulties in the bud once and for all.

But the outcome was far from what anyone expected.

Dr. Courcoulas couldn't perform the Roux-en-Y gastric bypass once I'd been opened on the operating table. She explained I had situs inversus - a rare condition where organs are reversed or mirrored from their normal positions.

Performing gastric bypass was not possible since my intestines faced the opposite direction. Dr. Courcoulas had located my otherwise healthy appendix on the lower *left* side of my abdomen and removed it as a precaution.

Long story short, what began as a gastric bypass operation ended up a $40,000 appendectomy.

Situs inversus is present in between one in 5,000 and one in 20,000 people in the United States, usually discovered during childhood. Since I never had surgery aside from wisdom tooth extraction, bunion removal and a corrective procedure for a minor foot bone deformity, the likelihood of situs inversus being discovered sooner was almost zero unless I'd developed appendicitis, which by the grace of God never happened.

My frustration level reached a point where I was about to resign myself to the fact I'd spend the rest of my life a huge blob ending up being unable to do virtually nothing for myself within a decade.

"God should issue a recall on me!" I blurted to a friend one afternoon. "Can someone find one thing *not* wrong for a change?"

"Well, He's kept you on Earth for some reason," he replied, "and Dr. Courcoulas recommended a laparoscopic adjustable band procedure during your post-op appointment."

"I'm not sure if I can deal with another year of jumping through hoops with more testing, another shrink exam, and battling the insurance company."

"What about all the times you expressed your worst fear of ending up like your mother? At least consider looking into a lap band."

She was right; I would have been crazy to pass up such an opportunity. Looking back, I'm glad I followed my friend's advice.

The second round of red tape didn't take long as the first. I passed the second psych evaluation and all other tests returned normal results.

I received a huge shock when the insurance carrier approved coverage of lap band surgery on my *first* effort!

Dr. Courcoulas' office planned surgery for mid-April 2007 at UPMC Magee-Women's Hospital, but unexpected changes moved my scheduled date to March 22 at eight in the morning. I remember little about the day until waking up following surgery.

"Well?" I groggily asked Dr. Courcoulas. "What's the verdict?"

"Everything went well. You'll be going to Recovery in a few minutes."

"You were able to put in the lap band?"

She gave me a broad smile. "It's in."

The last thing I remembered before falling asleep was pumping a fist in the air. After over two years of endless testing, dealing with insurance, failed gastric bypass, and other red tape, the long road to bariatric surgery finally came to an end.

***

The real work began after insertion of my lap band. I consumed nothing but ice chips the first twenty-four hours and began two weeks of clear liquids the following day. Another two weeks of full liquids were followed by two weeks on a soft diet before I resumed normal eating.

I'd like to say life after lap band surgery was perfect; unfortunately, that's not the case. I may not always adhere to the rules of a 1,100-calorie limit, especially during the holiday season.

On a positive note, I'm much thinner than I was ten years ago and can't recall the last time I dove into a full-blown binge.

The lap band is an incredible tool in further keeping my BED in check. Not only does it make me feel full sooner, but also a deterrent should I ever cave in to an urge to binge.

I once made the mistake of a "normal" over-indulgence during Thanksgiving dinner and spent the day's remainder bloated, cramped, and miserable. If a large holiday meal made me that uncomfortable, I can't begin to imagine how my old binge moments would feel nowadays!

There are many foods eaten over a lifetime I can no longer tolerate since having surgery, including several old "trigger" foods. I remind myself often to chew more thoroughly and eat slower, both key implements for lap band patients.

I'm still a long way from 150 pounds but have a full life remaining to reach my lofty goal. I still can't believe that a decade earlier I'd squeezed into size 30/32 and 5X plus size clothing, could barely walk on flat surfaces or stand longer than a few minutes without debilitating knee pain, had to sit to perform simple tasks such as dressing and seldom ventured out in public unless absolutely necessary.

If someone told me in 2004 that by 2014 I'd walk up and down hill sides with minor difficulty, have more good days than bad with my arthritis, complete house cleaning chores in less than two hours, dress in a standing position, shower without using a special seat, comfortably sit in armchairs, and buy clothes in a multitude of sizes ranging between plus sizes 18 and 22 and XL to 2X, I probably would've questioned their thinking.

Some limitations have remained; standing for more than a few hours and kneeling are still not plausible. My orthopedist stated even with present non-invasive treatment I'm currently receiving for arthritis- albeit successful thus far - knee replacement surgery will be needed in the future.

I can't work around dangerous machinery or in high places, drive a motor vehicle, climb ladders, or read anything smaller than eleven-point type, but I'm content with my impediments and attribute them to just getting older.

Considering all the physical and psychological turmoil weathered over a span of three decades, I can't help but think about the alternative outcomes if key decisions hadn't been made and appropriate treatments weren't feasible.

***

Practices and Benefits of Preventive Care

Preventive care are measures taken to prevent diseases and injuries in contrast to curing or treating symptoms. Consultations with medical professionals often come to mind when we hear the term "preventive care," but it involves more efforts on our part than believed.

Preventive care is usually tailored to an individual's age, overall health, and family history. A couple examples are regular prostate exams urged for men over 40 or someone at possible risk for diabetes having routine A1C (glycated hemoglobin) blood screenings, which measure plasma glucose concentration over extended periods of time.

Family history of certain cancers, heart disease, or other diseases sometimes warrant either increased frequency of health screenings or beginning regular tests earlier than recommended ages. In my case, while a Pap smear is needed only every two years, my gynecologist recommends checking my ovaries more often since there's a family history of ovarian cancer.

We should make health a top priority when sick or injured; otherwise we won't function at peak standard when in pain or feeling miserable. A plan for preventive care should be made far in advance and consistently practice healthy habits even during times employing preventive care inconveniences us. Simply put, maintaining healthy lifestyles are worth some sacrifices.

Finding and treating disease soon as possible are other important points in preventive care. We will eventually get sick, but when caught early, many diseases can be cured or symptoms brought under control to restore us to full health.

Becoming educated about illness, their symptoms, and what it takes to maintain overall good health work to our advantage. If detected soon enough, chances for a full recovery improve and most diseases becoming serious enough to affect our lifestyles with debilitating symptoms or death are abolished. Unfortunately, most health care systems are designated for treating illnesses and injuries once they've happened, such as trips to the emergency room for acute symptoms.

Many insurance plans cover routine office visits like physical exams, but preventive care is seldom main focus of the medical profession. Therefore, responsibility for making sure doctors understand an individual's personal goals of staying healthy and preventing disease being high priorities lie solely on us.

We should view preventive care as investments or insurance in our personal well-being. Take advantage of any preventive benefits your primary physician offers and are covered by insurance.

There are two clear-cut choices: we can either invest small amounts of time and money to maintain good health - some expenses are covered 100% by medical insurance - or pay massive out-of-pocket costs later to treat diseases and injuries that could happen. Since major medical expenses can easily exceed maximum insurance coverage, the latter comes with financial consequences, including bankruptcy.

Compare relatively inexpensive fees of regular check-ups against the enormous expenditures of major care such as cancer treatment or long-term skilled nursing care, all which can be reduced or prevented by utilizing preventive measures.

More people are beginning to make preventive care a focal point, thanks to increased awareness of its importance made by the media and easier access to crucial information.

Preventive care collectively benefits everyone by minimizing individual demands on the health care system and contributes to keeping the system efficient, affordable and smoothly functioning.

On the other hand, if too many people delay receiving treatment for illnesses and injuries, everyone's quality of health care suffers and medical expenses rise, resulting in higher costs, increased insurance premiums, poorer quality of service for each individual, and a highly-taxed medical system.

Preventive health care doesn't require a medical degree to be successful; using some common sense goes long way in preserving both our health and bank accounts. We can get a head start on our preventive care with the following:

- Don't smoke or use other tobacco products.

- Drink only in moderation or abstain from alcoholic beverages altogether.

- Eat a proper, well-balanced diet for correct daily amount of nutrients and calories.

- Exercise at least three days per week. You don't need to join a gym; brisk outdoor walks and home exercise programs are just as effective.

- See your doctor regularly for check-ups.

- Avoid using street drugs.

- Consume caffeinated products in moderation if you must have them at all.

- If you take prescription medication on a regular basis, adhere to prescribed dosages and become familiar with intended use, side effects, possible interactions with over-the-counter remedies and other prescriptions, and whether they can be taken with food or only on an empty stomach. *Never* lend or borrow prescription medication, as each is formulated toward individuals for whom they're prescribed.

- Drink plenty of water; 6-8 glasses daily are the usual recommended intake.

Take the time to learn more about preventive care and work on your healthy habits. While it takes considerable effort to break bad habits such as smoking, building good ones requires little time. I guarantee you will thank yourselves sometime in the near future by becoming healthier, more energetic and enjoying life to its fullest.

***

Preventive care isn't limited to our bodies; strong psychological well-being and sharp minds are also important to overall good health. Preventive care to reduce and stave off physical symptoms may be a no-brainer among many, but it's surprising how few people partake in activities beneficial to cognitive clarity and psychological advantages.

Luminosity.com emphasizes "brain training." Many of you have probably seen television commercials or spotted ads on various Internet web sites for Luminosity and wondered how some of the site's features could benefit you.

Luminosity aims to develop personalized training programs to build strength in memory, attention, speed, flexibility and problem solving. The joy of Luminosity's brain exercises is that they have a feel of playing online games; you can keep key areas of the mind keen while having fun doing it.

Reading, crossword puzzles, creative writing, art and craft projects, assembling jigsaw puzzles, model building (ships, cars, airplanes, etc.), musical pursuits, playing board games, and wood working are other examples of activities that can keep the mind active while producing personal enjoyment.

Preventive psychological care is important as the physical aspects; if we neglect one, chances are good the other suffers. Of all known psychological afflictions, stress appears to be the most common denominator among people from all walks of life.

Did you know 85% of all illnesses are related to stress? According to the World Health Organization, the number one global epidemic is stress. In other words, stress can kill!

It's normal to have certain degrees of stress in our lives, but elevated levels can have impacts on both physical and psychological well-being. When overwhelmed by stress, we tend to do things like make poor decisions, overeat or not eat at all, engage in drug use, compulsive shopping or unprotected sex with multiple partners, easily lose our tempers, and yes, develop symptoms of physical ailments.

The American Psychological Association published findings on physical and psychological reactions to stress in men and women. Both genders manage stress in markedly different ways; while men experience their fair share of stress, women are more likely to report stress-related physical symptoms.

Some of American Psychological Association's findings included:

- Women are more likely than men to report that their stress levels are on the rise. They are also much more likely than men to report physical and emotional symptoms of stress. When comparing women with each other, there also appears to be differences in the ways that married and single women experience stress.

- Women are more likely than men (28 percent vs. 20 percent) to report having a great deal of stress (8, 9 or 10 on a 10-point scale). Almost half of all women (49 percent) surveyed said their stress has increased over the past five years, compared to four in 10 (39 percent) men. Women are more likely to report that money (79 percent compared with 73 percent of men) and the economy (68 percent compared with 61 percent of men) are sources of stress while men are far more likely to cite that work is a source of stress (76 percent compared with 65 percent of women).

- Married women report higher levels of stress than single women, with one-third (33 percent) reporting that they have experienced a great deal of stress in the past month (8, 9 or 10 on a 10-point scale) compared with one in five (22 percent) of single women. Similarly, significantly more married women report that their stress has increased over the past five years (56 percent vs. 41 percent of single women). Single women are also more likely than married women to say they feel they are doing enough to manage their stress (63 percent vs. 51 percent). Married women are more likely than single women to report they have experienced the following due to stress in the past month: feeling as though they could cry (54 percent vs. 33 percent), feeling irritable or angry (52 percent vs. 38 percent), having headaches (48 percent vs. 33 percent) and experiencing fatigue (47 percent vs. 35 percent). Men and women report wide gaps between determining what is important and how successful they are at achieving those behaviors.

- Women are much more likely than men to say that having a good relationship with their families is important to them (84 percent vs. 74 percent). While fewer women say they are doing a good job at succeeding in this area, they outpace men (67 percent vs. 53 percent).

- Women are also more likely than men to say that having a good relationship with their friends is important to them (69 percent vs. 62 percent), even though friendship is cited less often than family for both men and women. Even though nearly half of all women (49 percent) say they have lain awake at night in the past month because of stress, three-quarters of women rate getting enough sleep as extremely or very important (75 percent compared with 58 percent of men).

- Across the board, men's and women's perceptions of their ability to succeed in areas that are important to their well-being are far out of line with the importance they place on these behaviors. Even more so than women, men report less likelihood of success in these areas.

- Only 33 percent of women report being successful in their efforts to get enough sleep (compared with 75 percent who believe this is important); only 35 percent report success in their efforts to manage stress (compared with 69 percent who believe this is important); 36 percent report success in their efforts to eat healthy (compared with 64 percent who believe this is important); and only 29 percent are successful in their efforts to be physically active (compared with 54 percent who believe this is important).

- Only 25 percent of men report being successful in their efforts to get enough sleep (compared with 58 percent who believe this is important); only 30 percent report success in their efforts to manage stress (compared with 59 percent who believe this is important); only 25 percent report success in their efforts to eat healthy (compared with 52 percent who believe this is important); and only 26 percent are successful in their efforts to be physically active (compared with 54 percent who believe this is important).

No matter what our gender, in order to deal with stress, find peace of mind and untangle life's knots, we should take steps to relax more so we can tune in to our bodies' own wisdom.

The American Heart Association offers four simple yet stress coping techniques that can be applied almost anywhere:

- **Self-talk.** We all talk to ourselves; sometimes we talk out loud but usually in our heads. Self-talk can be positive or negative. Negative self-talk increases stress while positive self-talk helps calm us and control stress. With practice, we can learn to turn negative thoughts into positive ones.

- **Emergency Stress Stoppers.** We endure many stressful situations - at work, home, on the road and public places. We may feel stress because of poor communication, too much work and everyday hassles like standing in line. Emergency stress stoppers help you deal with stress on the spot; for example, counting to ten before speaking or taking three to five deep breaths.

- **Finding pleasure.** When stress makes us feel bad, we should do something that makes us feel good. Doing things we enjoy is a natural way to fight off stress. Even when we're depressed or sick, we can find pleasure in simple things such as going for a drive, chatting with a friend or reading a good book. Try to do at least one enjoyable thing daily, even if it's only for 15 minutes.

- **Daily relaxation.** Relaxation is more than sitting in a favorite chair watching TV. To relieve stress, relaxation should calm the tension in mind and body. Some good forms of relaxation are yoga, tai chi (a series of slow, graceful movements) and meditation. Deep breathing is also a form of relaxation and can easily be learned at home.

Stress is inevitable; when it strikes, it can feel like you're attacked from every angle. That's why having healthy tools to coping tools are important. Having solid plans to prevent and handle stress can make a difference between quickly extinguishing a minor emotional brush fire and experiencing a three-alarm meltdown.

***

Whether your concerns lie in keeping your diabetes under control or discovering new ways to live a better life despite a mental health diagnosis, it's safe to think all of us agree on the importance of preventive care.

When we adopt the mentality that doctors can't help everyone improve their health - there aren't enough hours in each day - it will become easier to take the initiative needed to make needed inner and outer health changes.

We owe it to ourselves and loved ones to be in the best health possible; therefore, we should make preventative care a priority in America. Are you ready to accept the challenge of being in charge of your good health?

***

Resources

We all know preventing disease and maximizing personal health are two essential activities of a well-functioning and prolonged life span, but another aspect of preventive care is finding additional options through non-profit and other organizations focusing on prevention and treatment of various diseases and disorders.

Such organizations offer a wide spectrum of information to the public ranging from printed educational materials, Internet web sites to free and low cost services, advocacy, and - in some cases - full or partial financial assistance for essential medical procedures not covered by insurance.

I utilized some resources while undergoing various types medical treatment; others I explored while writing this book. Many I list in this chapter expand throughout the nation or worldwide while others only operate in certain regions.

Organizations listed on the following pages include both non-profit and others dedicated to health and well-being.

***

NON-PROFIT ORGANIZATIONS

American Cancer Society
http://www.cancer.org
Phone: (800) 227-2345

The American Cancer Society has led the way to transform cancer from deadly to preventable for 100 years.

American Heart Association
http://www.heart.org
Phone:
(800) 242-8721
(888) 474-VIVE

The American Heart Association is a non-profit organization in the United States that fosters appropriate cardiac care in an effort to reduce disability and deaths caused by cardiovascular disease and stroke. The American Heart Association also offers CPR and first aid courses.

American Sleep Apnea Association
http://www.sleepapnea.org
Phone: (888) 293-3650
Fax: (888) 293-3650

Founded in 1990, the American Sleep Apnea Association (ASAA) promotes awareness of sleep apnea, works for continuing improvements in treatments for this serious disease, and advocates for the interests of sleep apnea patients. ASAA also offers a CPAP Assistance program, which offers gently used CPAPs in order to put them in the hands of those who need therapy but don't have the means to pay for it or insurance that provides coverage.

Arthritis Foundation
http://www.arthritis.org
National Office: (404) 872-7100

The Arthritis Foundation's mission is to improve lives through leadership in the prevention, control and cure of arthritis and related diseases. Their vision is to create a world free of arthritis pain.

The Breast Cancer Site - GreaterGood
http://thebreastcancersite.greatergood.com
University Street, Suite 1000
Seattle, WA 98101-4107

The Breast Cancer Site was founded to help fund free mammograms for women in need - women for whom early detection would not otherwise be possible. Since its launch in October 2000, the site has established itself as a leader in online activism and in the fight to prevent breast cancer deaths.

Crisis Center of Tampa Bay
http://www.crisiscenter.com
One Crisis Center Plaza
Tampa, FL 33613-1238
(813) 964-1964

The Crisis Center of Tampa Bay help those in need deal with devastating traumas of sexual assault or abuse, domestic violence, financial distress, substance abuse, medical emergencies, suicidal thoughts, emotional or situational problems. The Crisis Center of Tampa Bay is available 24 hours 365 days a year.

Epilepsy Foundation of America
http://www.epilepsyfoundation.org
Phone: 1-800-332-1000

The Epilepsy Foundation of America® is the national voluntary health agency dedicated solely to the welfare of the more than 2 million people with epilepsy in the U.S. and their families.

Health Foundation of South Florida
http://hfsf.org
Phone: (305) 374-7200
Fax: (305) 374-7003

The Health Foundation of South Florida's mission is to improve the health of people residing in Broward, Miami-Dade and Monroe Counties. By funding providers and supporting programs to promote health and prevent disease, HFSF makes measurable and sustainable differences in the health of individuals and families.

Highmark Health
https://www.highmarkhealth.org
Fifth Avenue Place
Fifth Avenue
Pittsburgh, PA 15222-3099
Phone: (412) 544-7000

Highmark Health's mission is to make high quality health care easily accessible, understandable and affordable, with a vision to be recognized leader in structuring, financing and delivering high quality and affordable health care.

NAMI: National Alliance on Mental Illness
http://www.nami.org
Phone: (703) 524-7600
Fax: (703) 524-9094
Member Services: (888) 999-6264

NAMI is the nation's largest grassroots mental health organization dedicated to building better lives for the millions of Americans affected by mental illness. NAMI advocates for access to services, treatment, supports and research and is steadfast in its commitment to raise awareness and build a community for hope for all of those in need.

National Eating Disorders Association
http://www.nationaleatingdisorders.org
Information and Referrals: (800) 931-2237
Email: info@NationalEatingDisorders.org

The National Eating Disorders Association (NEDA) is the leading non-profit organization in the United States advocating on behalf and supporting individuals and families affected by eating disorders campaigning for prevention, improved access to quality treatment, and increased research funding to better understand and treat eating disorders.

National Suicide Prevention Hotline
http://www.suicidepreventionlifeline.org
Phone: (800) 273-8255

The National Suicide Prevention Lifeline is a 24-hour, toll-free, confidential suicide prevention hotline available to anyone in suicidal crisis or emotional distress. By dialing 1-800-273-TALK (8255), the call is routed to the nearest crisis center in our national network of more than 150 crisis centers. The Lifeline's national network of local crisis centers provides crisis counseling and mental health referrals day and night.

Obesity Action Coalition
http://www.obesityaction.org
North Himes Avenue
Tampa, FL 33614
(813) 872-7835

The Obesity Action Coalition (OAC) is a nearly 50,000 member-strong organization dedicated to giving a voice to the individual affected by the disease of obesity and helping individuals along their journey toward better health through education, advocacy and support.

The Starkey Hearing Foundation Hear Now Program
http://www.starkeyhearingfoundation.org/programs/hear-now
Phone: (866) 354-3254

Hear Now is committed to assisting U.S. residents with hearing loss, who have no resources to acquire hearing aids. Starkey Hearing Foundation provides the hearing aids and runs the program, but count on the generosity of Hear Now providers and donors across the country to ensure its success.

Susan G. Komen
http://ww5.komen.org
Phone: (877) 465-6636

Since 1982, Susan G. Komen has played a critical role in every major advance in the fight against breast cancer, transforming how the world talks about and treats this disease and helping to turn millions of breast cancer patients into breast cancer survivors.

University of Pittsburgh Medical Center (UPMC)
http://www.upmc.com
Lothrop Street
Pittsburgh, PA 15213-2582
Phone: (800)533-8762

University of Pittsburgh Medical Center (UPMC) is a $10 billion integrated global nonprofit health enterprise that has 54,000 employees, 20 hospitals, 4,733 licensed beds, 400 outpatient sites and doctors' offices, a 2.2 million-member health insurance division, as well as commercial and international ventures.

***

ADDITIONAL RESOURCES

Anita P. Courcoulas, M.D., MPH, F A.C.S.
UPMC Magee-Womens Hospital
Halket Street, Suite 5600
Pittsburgh, PA 15213
Phone: (412) 641-3632

Dr. Anita Courcoulas is a bariatric and general surgeon at Magee-Womens Hospital of UPMC. She received her undergraduate degree at Brown University and her medical degree from Boston University School of Medicine.

She completed her surgical training at the University of Pittsburgh Medical Center, along with advanced training in pediatric, trauma, and minimally invasive surgery. She specializes in the laparoscopic approach to treat obesity and other diseases of the foregut. Dr. Courcoulas' particular areas of interest include the surgical treatment of massive obesity, gastroesophageal reflux disease and obesity, and the cancer risks of obesity.

Dr. Courcoulas has published and authored over 50 articles, book chapters, and reviews related to pediatric, trauma, bariatric, and minimally invasive surgery. She is a committed teacher and has lectured extensively across the United States on a variety of subjects related to her fields of expertise.

Lakewood Psychiatric Hospital
342 Linden Creek Road
Canonsburg, PA 15317
Phone: (724) 746-2400

Lakewood Psychiatric Hospital is a 21-bed facility providing short-term inpatient treatment.

Menninger Clinic
http://www.menningerclinic.com
Phone: (800) 351-9058

Menninger Clinic is one of the nation's leading inpatient psychiatric hospitals dedicated to treating individuals with complex mental illness, including severe mood, personality, anxiety and addictive disorders.

National Institute of Mental Health
http://www.nimh.nih.gov
Phone: (866) 615-6464
Email: nimhinfo@nih.gov

The mission of NIMH is to transform the understanding and treatment of mental illnesses through basic and clinical research, paving the way for prevention, recovery, and cure.

ObesityHelp
http://www.obesityhelp.com
Phone: (866) 957-4636

ObesityHelp was founded in 1998 as a peer support community to help those faced with life threatening morbid obesity. By June of 1999, the site's existence has been brought to the attention of clinicians and professionals and the organization was formalized to extend support to patients and clinicians while expanding the scope of its public outreach activities. ObesityHelp's web site has over 3,000,000 page-views a week from people looking for help.

Overeaters Anonymous
http://www.oa.org
Phone: (505) 891-2664
Fax: (505) 891-4320

Overeaters Anonymous is a Fellowship of individuals who, through shared experience, strength and hope, are recovering from compulsive overeating. OA welcomes everyone who wants to stop eating compulsively. There are no dues or fees for members; OA is self-supporting through their own contributions, neither soliciting nor accepting outside donations. OA is not affiliated with any public or private organization, political movement, ideology or religious doctrine; they take no position on outside issues.

The Juicy Woman
http://www.thejuicywoman.com
Brave People International
dba The Juicy Woman
P.O. Box 576
Nanuet, NY 10954-0576
Phone: (845) 425-1661

Best resource on the Web to create daily confidence; make peace with food and behavioral learning tools such as Emotional Freedom Technique (EFT) to love the skin you're in.

Twin Lakes Center
http://www.twinlakescenter.org
Twin Lakes Road
Somerset, PA 15501
Phone: (800) 452-0218

Twin Lakes Center has provided drug and alcohol rehabilitation services since 1983. The main campus is located on over 30 acres of land in rural Somerset County, PA. The remote but easily accessible location provides a quiet and relaxing, recovery environment. Services at the main campus include detoxification, short term residential treatment, partial hospitalization, outpatient and intensive outpatient treatment.

Veterans Health Administration
http://www.va.gov/health
Veterans Crisis Line: (800) 273-8255 (press 1)

The Veterans Health Administration is America's largest integrated health care system with over 1,700 sites of care, serving 8.76 million veterans each year.

***

Acknowledgments

Of course, it's been said many times before: without the key people making respective effects on my life, I'd never had motivation to write this book.

I am forever grateful for the love and support provided to me by those who inspired me to keep pushing forward, whether to not give up finding concrete answers to health issues or continue pursuing my dreams: nieces Lisa Mounts-McGrath and Deidre Dennick-Seibert; nephew-in-law Mark McGrath, friends Sister Bernadette Schaad, Shelly Dechert, Dawn Lilly, Jennifer Patuleia-Duffy and her husband Brian Duffy, Matt Hoover, Anthony Piers, Mindy Robbins and her boyfriend Micheal Workman, Greg McNeish, Mike Siciliano, Anthony Valvo, Samantha Wallace, Martha Montufar, the gang at Steel City Buzz, and Donovan (Don) Rutherford, personal manager, sounding board, and love of my life.

How could I go without acknowledging those in the medical profession assisting in planning my preventive care goals and who diagnosed, treated, and caught abnormalities in early stages? I'll keep it simple: thanks to Dr. Rudolph Antoncic, Jr. and nurses of Health First Medical Associates and Dr. Michael Tranovich and his staff at Pittsburgh Bone and Joint.

I'm much obliged to Dr. Anita Courcoulas and Amy Drusak, PA-C of UPMC Magee-Womens Minimally Invasive and Bariatric Surgery, Dr. Robert Simmonds of Womancare Associates; Dr. Patrick J. Strollo, Jr. of the UPMC Sleep Medicine Center, Mark Gustina, MS CCC-A and Lucinda Swallow of Cranberry Hearing and Balance, Dr. Neil Hart of Frazier-Hart Cardiovascular and his former associates Dr. John Paulowski and Dr. John Wilson for their dedication to my health care.

Special thanks to hospitals and miscellaneous health care agencies for their tireless efforts to provide quality care and resources for patients: UPMC McKeesport, UPMC Montifore, UPMC Magee-Women's, UPMC Mercy, UPMC Shadyside, UPMC Presbyterian, UPMC Western Psychiatric Institute and Clinic, Allegheny General Hospital, The Washington Hospital, Lakewood Psychiatric Hospital, Menninger Clinic, Sandin Home Health, the research staff of Longitudinal Assessment of Bariatric Surgery (LABS), Edward Grandi of the American Sleep Apnea Association, the Arthritis Foundation Central & Western Pennsylvania chapter, Susan G. Komen, and Office of Rare Diseases at the National Institute of Health.

I cannot forget colleagues who share victories and defeats that come with being authors: Kristal McKerrington, Danielle Zwissler, Lorraine Holloway-White, Shelly Ramm, Andrea Amador, Stacey Danson, Jessica Degarmo, Shannon Lee, Sessha Batto, Tee Geering, Jillian Ward, Johnnie McCoy, George Polley, Tim and Kathleen Hewston, Poppet, Lily Byrne, Shonell Bacon, Diane Nelson, Gerry and Raymond McCullough, Lynette Carrington (no relation), Jamie Saloff, Brie Tate, Joanne Ellis, Kelle Groom, Kate Rigby, Gary Ponzo, Stella Deluze, K.J. Kron, Tallulah Rose, C.K. Webb, Mat Jackson, Loretta Proctor, Paul Freeman, Charity Parkerson, Bobby Hilliard, Randy Attwood, Shelia Mary Belshaw, John Booth, Splinker Smityh, Shalini Boland, Simon Swift, Christine Schwab, Lisa Scottoline, and Barbara Bentley.

A shout out to people who inspire me to keep the creative energies flowing: Peter Gruner, Joe E. Legend, Brian Kendrick, Stacy Hunter, Pete Gasparino, Lacey Adkisson, Pete Sisseam, TJ Wilson, Adrian Lionheart McCallum, Goldy Locks, Diana Hart Smith, and Billy Silverman. I hope to someday personally meet all of you, whether again or for the first time.

Publishers and organizations that deserve recognition for bringing many talented independent authors into the spotlight: Turning the Pages Books, Night Owl Reviews, Coffee Time Romance & More, Page Readers, Authors on Show, The Polka Dot Banner, Pennwriters, National Novel Writing Month (NaNoWriMo), Oosa Book Club, Goodreads, She Writes, The Independent Author Network, AuthorsDB, American Society for Journalists and Authors, Indie Gypsy, Firefly & Wisp Books, Wild Child Publishing, Romance Writers of America, WebbWeaver Books, and WOW!(Women on Writing).

Additional gratitude is extended to those working behind the scenes of my publishers, Palm Tree Books and That Right Publishing/Taylor Street Books. Their dedication has not gone unnoticed.

Finally, thank you to all my readers; you are the ones who make what is sometimes a difficult job worthwhile.

About the Author

L. Anne Carrington is an Amazon bestselling author, freelance writer/journalist, and radio show host whose previous work covered topics from fiction to news stories, human interest features, and entertainment reviews. She wrote *The Wrestling Babe* Internet column for seven years, a former music reviewer for *Indie Music Stop*, former book reviewer for Free Press (an imprint of Simon and Schuster), and pens several other works which appears in both print and Web media.

One of her freelance articles, *An Overview of Causes of Hearing Loss and Deafness,* was bought by Internet Broadcasting Systems, a company that co-produced NBCOlympics.com for the 2004 Summer Olympics in Athens and the 2006 Torino Winter Olympics in addition to being the leading provider of Web sites, content and advertising revenue solutions to the largest and most successful media companies.

In addition to her acclaimed novels in *The Cruiserweight Series* among works of both fiction and nonfiction, Ms. Carrington hosts *The L. Anne Carrington Show* on Spreaker Radio Wednesdays at 2:00 PM Eastern.

She spends time between Pittsburgh, PA and Tampa, FL, continuing to write.

www.ingramcontent.com/pod-product-compliance
Lightning Source LLC
Chambersburg PA
CBHW050550280326
41933CB00011B/1795